Restorative Yoga

A Healing Mind-Body Practice for Managing Chronic Illness

Table of Contents

Chapter 1. Introduction

Journey with us as we delve into the serene and healing world of Restorative Yoga in this exclusive Special Report. Discover an oasis of calm amidst the challenge of chronic illness, where each breath brings respite and every pose heals - not just the body, but the mind and the spirit as well. Unfold the science behind its therapeutic effects, and hear from proponents who have regained their health and vitality. This transformative practice could be the missing key in your management of chronic illness, offering a sanctuary from the storm. We invite you to explore the rejuvenating experience that Restorative Yoga offers, affirming that relief is within your reach, and resilience, within you. Let this Special Report guide you towards a journey of restoration, serenity, and healing that springs from within.

Chapter 2. A Gentle Introduction to Restorative Yoga

Restorative Yoga, a unique offshoot of traditional yoga, utilizes props to make yoga poses unchallenging, accommodating, and comfortable. These props may include yoga bolsters, blocks, blankets, and straps, used by practitioners to support the body in ways that foster maximum relaxation and wellness.

"Restorative" is derived from the Latin word "restaurare," which means to renew or restore. As the name implies, Restorative Yoga aims to restore harmony between the body, mind, and spirit. Practitioners embark on a journey of relaxation, rejuvenation, and restoration that transcends the physical body to elevate the spirit and calm the mind.

2.1. Origins of Restorative Yoga

The genesis of Restorative Yoga can be traced back to B.K.S. Iyengar, a highly influential yogi from India. He invented the use of props in yoga to make it more accessible and beneficial for all, regardless of age, flexibility or physical condition. Iyengar's student, Judith Hanson Lasater, is largely credited with popularizing Restorative Yoga in the West.

Restorative Yoga was established on the philosophy that passive relaxation can trigger the parasympathetic nervous system, which commands the body's rest-and-digest response. Being more in tune with this response allows the body and mind to relax deeply, inducing a state of profound tranquility.

2.2. How Does Restorative Yoga Work?

Every and each pose in Restorative Yoga is meticulously constructed to place least possible physical stress on the body. The use of props allows for a level of comfort which encourages the body to fully surrender into poses, promoting a sense of deep relaxation. For many, Restorative Yoga poses are reminiscent of lounging, reclining, or resting in a comfortable position.

The emphasis here is less on performing the poses to perfection, but more on achieving a sense of comfort and relaxation. Postures are usually held for an extended period, typically five to twenty minutes.

2.3. Mind-Body Connection

Arguably the most transformative aspect of Restorative Yoga lies in its potential to enhance the connection between the body and the mind. As the body learns to rest, release tension and surrender to the pose, the mind follows suit. This gradual itinerary towards relaxation fosters mindfulness and encourages individuals to pay heed to their breath, sensations, thoughts, and emotions.

Moreover, the heartbeat slows, the respiratory rate decreases, and the body cools down - a state mimicking that of deep sleep. It promotes healing and regeneration, both physiologically and psychologically. It is not uncommon for practitioners to experience emotional release, often attributing a sense of peace and tranquility to regular practice.

2.4. Benefits of Restorative Yoga

Restorative Yoga's comprehensive approach to wellness has a wide array of benefits. These not only address physical ailments but also alleviate psychological and emotional distress.

Table 1. Benefits of Restorative Yoga

Physical Benefits	Psychological Benefits
Enhances Flexibility	Reduces Stress and Anxiety
Improves Capacity for Deeper Breathing	Encourages Mindfulness
Balances the Nervous System	Alleviates Depression
Boosts Immune System	Improves Concentration and Mood

Knowing that it caters to total well-being makes Restorative Yoga an attractive choice for those seeking for holistic healing, or simply for a sanctuary of calm amidst the upheaval of modern living. Chronic illness sufferers often find solace and relief in the comforting envelope of Restorative Yoga.

2.5. The Practice of Restorative Yoga

Before you embark on this yoga journey, remember that success in Restorative Yoga lies not in achieving the perfect pose, but in achieving the feeling of relaxation and rejuvenation at the end of each practice. Each pose is adjustable and should be tailored to your body's specific needs and comfort levels.

Here are some commonly performed Restorative poses:

1. Child's Pose (Balasana)

2. Reclining Bound Angle Pose (Supta Baddha Konasana)

3. Legs-Up-The-Wall Pose (Viparita Karani)

4. Reclining Hero Pose (Supta Virasana)

2.6. Conclusion

Restorative Yoga is your ally in coping with the rigors of chronic illness, stress, and modern life. It rejuvenates your vital energy, making you better equipped to handle the pressures of life. It offers a reprieve without demanding physical strength or flexibility. The holistic spirit of healing in Restorative Yoga is something that everyone can embrace, as it believes in the power of the self, and the tranquility that evolves from within.

Embrace this practice willingly and you'll discover the profound impact Restorative Yoga can have on your physical, emotional, and spiritual well-being. The sanctuary of calm you seek is within reach; it begins and ends with you.

Chapter 3. Decoding the Mind-Body Connection

The mysteries of the human mind and body connection are awe-inspiring. Restorative Yoga, renowned for its ability to restore and rejuvenate the practitioner, serves as a tool in uncovering these mysteries. Our journey in this chapter begins with understanding the body's stress-response system and the role it plays in chronic illnesses. We then dive deeper into the sea of restorative yoga's effect on stress reduction and how exactly this practice speaks to our body and mind.

3.1. The Body's Stress-Response System

The stress-response mechanism of the body, also known as the "fight or flight" response, kicks into high gear in response to perceived threats. Whether it's an urgent deadline or a predator on the prowl, the body's systems respond identically: pulse quickens, breath shortens, muscles tense, and adrenaline rushes through the bloodstream. The body, preparing for a rigorous physical response, puts on hold the non-emergency processes such as digestion or immune response. This is survival mode.

However, our modern lives trap us in a prolonged state of this "fight or flight" response, leading to a chronic stress condition that spirals into a plethora of health complications, ranging from cardiovascular diseases to depression and anxiety disorders. Chronic stress disrupts the body's equilibrium, and herein lies the core of numerous chronic ailments.

3.2. Restorative Yoga and Stress Reduction

From this point of understanding, we turn to restorative yoga - a soothing balm for the body trapped in chronic stress mode. Restorative yoga promotes relaxation, encouraging the body to shift from the stress-propelled "fight or flight" response to the rest-and-digest system, our body's mode of healing and restoration.

Restorative yoga targets the parasympathetic nervous system, the element of our nervous system that governs rest, digestion, and healing. Through its deep, measured breaths and gentle, supported poses, this practice nudges the body into a state of deep relaxation and healing.

Regular practice inverses the stress response, calming your heart rate, lowering blood pressure, and enhancing digestion. This creates a nurturing environment for your body to repair tissues and cells, nullifying the effects of prolonged stress and chronic illnesses.

3.3. How Restorative Yoga Speaks to the Body and Mind

Understanding the connection between stress and chronic illness paves the way to appreciate how restorative yoga unifies mind and body to promote healing. Every element in a restorative yoga class—the subdued lighting, peaceful ambiance, slow tempo, and gentle poses—murmur in unison: it is time to relax.

Let's listen to what happens next. From the first inhalation and stretch, your body begins to launch its natural restorative processes. Internal organs that had been primed for action under stress are now relaxing and rejuvenating. Blood flow is rerouted to depleted areas to repair and restore balance.

The pose does not merely shape your body but also your mind. Every pose is an active embodiment of mindfulness. As you maintain a pose, you are encouraged to draw your attention to your breath and the sensations pulsing within your body. This ushers in a meditative state of mind, clearing the cobwebs of anxiety and stress, thereby bringing mental clarity and calm.

Psychological studies report a noticeable reduction in stress, anxiety, and depressive symptoms among regular practitioners of restorative yoga. Plus, the enhanced self-awareness and mindfulness aid in intercepting stress-inducing thought patterns, equipping you with the ability to manage your stress response better.

3.4. The Ripple Effect of Healing

As we navigate the intricacies of restorative yoga and its effects on the body and mind, we begin to comprehend its potential beyond immediate, personal healing. Regular practice forms a ripple of wellness that extends outwards from the practitioner. When you are healed, serene, and mentally robust, it reflects in everything you do and everyone you encounter - from your interpersonal relationships to your productivity at work.

In summary, restorative yoga's therapeutic effect stems from its potential to reduce stress and facilitate the body's innate healing processes. Seeing it not just as a physical form of exercise, but rather a series of mindful movements that calm the mind and invigorate the body, reveals its holistic healing potential. This practice may indeed be a crucial key for many on their journey towards managing chronic illness and restoring their health. So unfurl your yoga mat, let your breath guide your movements as you commence on a path towards balance, serenity, and wellness.

Chapter 4. Unlocking Restorative Yoga: Postures and Props

Restorative yoga is a gentle form of yoga that promotes relaxation, calm, and healing in the body. It uses a variety of props, from bolsters to blankets, blocks, straps, and eye pillows, which enable the practitioner to hold poses for longer periods, offering the body an opportunity to sink deeper into relaxation and restoration. The postures, combined with a controlled breathing technique and meditative mindset, provide a holistic approach to stress relief and healing.

4.1. Understanding the Magic of Restorative Yoga

At its core, restorative yoga emphasizes the importance of relaxation and rest. In today's fast-paced world, stress has become a common element in many people's lives, leading to chronic illnesses and mental health conditions. Restorative yoga offers an oasis where one can disconnect from the mundane demands and surrender the mind, body, and Soul to a peaceful state.

This practice utilizes postures designed to open the body in passive and gentle ways. The strategic placement of props supports the body as it eases into relaxation and release. Unlike active yoga styles where movements are fluid and constant, in restorative yoga, practitioners enter a pose and stay there for an extended period. This stillness creates a conducive environment for mental clarity and calm to seep in.

4.2. The Science Behind Restorative Yoga

Modern science supports the benefits of restorative yoga. Research suggests that this practice can activate the parasympathetic nervous system, which controls our body's rest and digest functions. This activation leads to slower heart rates, lower blood pressure, and a decrease in stress hormones, thus promoting healing and rejuvenation.

Moreover, restorative yoga encourages mindfulness, deep relaxation, and a meditation-like state, resulting in improved mood, better sleep, and a sense of overall wellbeing. The mind-body connection attained through this practice offers a unique and holistic approach to managing chronic illnesses by reducing both physical and emotional symptoms.

4.3. The Transformative Postures

Restorative Yoga revolves around a set of specific postures aimed at relaxation and restoration. Although these poses might appear simple, they carry extraordinary healing power. Following are some of the key postures used in restorative yoga:

- Savasana (Corpse Pose): This pose involves lying flat on the back, legs slightly apart and arms relaxed beside the body. It allows complete relaxation of the body, releasing physical and mental tension.

- Balasana (Child's Pose): This is a deeply relaxing pose that stretches the lower back, hips, thighs, and ankles, while calming the mind and relieving stress and tension.

- Supta Baddha Konasana (Reclining Bound Angle Pose): This reclining pose helps open the hips and chest. It can provide relief from symptoms of menopause, mild depression, and insomnia.

- Viparita Karani (Legs-Up-The-Wall Pose): This pose involves lying on the back with legs resting against a wall. It relieves tired leg muscles, reduces swelling in the feet, and calms the nervous system.

4.4. The Role of Props in Restorative Yoga

Props are essential in restorative yoga as they provide comfort, support, stability, and alignment in the poses. They help cushion the body, allowing it to open up through passive stretching. Here are some commonly used props and their functions:

- Yoga Bolsters: They are firm pillows used to support the body, reduce strain on the muscles and promote deep relaxation.

- Yoga Blocks: These are used to help bring the floor closer, making poses more accessible. They can provide support to the hands, hips, or feet, depending on the pose.

- Yoga Straps: These are used to help extend reach and improve flexibility. They can be utilized in poses where the hands don't easily meet, such as in the seated forward bend.

- Yoga Blankets: They provide warmth, comfort, and extra padding. They can also be used to elevate the hips in seated poses or support the neck and back.

- Yoga Eye Pillows: They help to soothe the eyes and the mind, promoting deep relaxation and an internal focus.

With its emphasis on complete relaxation, restorative yoga is a valuable practice for managing stress responses and achieving mental, emotional, and physical balance. It shows us that we don't always have to push hard or strive for more – sometimes, the most profound changes can come when we allow ourselves the space and time to just be. Whether you're coping with a chronic illness or simply the stresses of daily life, the postures and props of restorative yoga can prove transformative on your journey to wellness.

Chapter 5. The Science Behind Restorative Yoga

Restorative Yoga, aptly named given its ability to restore the body and the mind, is a practice grounded in science. Yoga has been a therapeutic tool employed by many to manage and alleviate a wide range of chronic illnesses and conditions. Let's delve into what science has to say about it.

5.1. The Core Tenet of Restorative Yoga

At its very core, Restorative Yoga promotes relaxation. Unlike other forms of exercise that necessitate exertion, Restorative Yoga is based on the principle of relaxation and rest, of surrendering to gravity and yielding to the support of props. This allows for complete relaxation, facilitating the release of physical and mental tension to promote healing.

The "Relaxation Response" developed by Dr. Herbert Benson of Harvard Medical School reinforces the science behind this core principle. Dr. Benson discovered that a series of physiological changes, termed the "relaxation response," could be elicited through various relaxation practices, Yoga being one of them. This response counters the stress or "fight or flight" response and activates the body's parasympathetic nervous system, often referred to as the rest and digest system, culminating in a range of positive health effects including lowered heart rate, blood pressure, and cortisol levels.

5.2. The Neurological Effect

Restorative Yoga, with its focus on rest and relaxation, has significant neurological effects that contribute to its healing power. When the body is relaxed and stress levels are minimized, the brain functions more effectively. This formulates the basis of the neurological perspective on Restorative Yoga.

Brain-derived neurotrophic factor (BDNF), a protein that supports and promotes the health of brain cells, plays a significant role in the effect Restorative Yoga has on the nervous system. Regularly practicing Restorative Yoga enhances BDNF levels. Higher BDNF levels are associated with better brain health, stress management, and emotion regulation.

Restorative Yoga also increases GABA (gamma-aminobutyric acid) levels. Low levels of GABA have been linked to anxiety and depression. In a study conducted by Dr. Chris Streeter, it was discovered that a consistent Yoga and meditation practice increased GABA levels which correlated with reduced anxiety and improved mood.

5.3. The Immune Response and Chronic Inflammation

Chronic inflammation, caused by prolonged stress and unhealthy lifestyle habits, has been linked to a variety of illnesses such as heart disease and diabetes. Restorative Yoga, working through the stress pathway, can help manage this inflammation and thereby combat these illnesses.

Restorative Yoga exercises have a significant positive effect on the functional capacity of the immune system. These practices reduce the secretion of stress hormones, which can suppress the immune response. A study by the Ohio State University found that women who routinely practiced Yoga had lower levels of the inflammatory cytokine TNF-alpha, demonstrating an immune-boosting effect.

5.4. Hormonal Effects

Restorative Yoga also has profound impacts on the body's hormonal balance. Cortisol, often known as the stress hormone, can wreak havoc on the body when its levels are unregulated. Restorative Yoga, with its focus on relaxation and mindfulness, helps to manage cortisol levels.

In chronic stress conditions, high cortisol levels may lead to mood disorders, weight gain, and even more serious conditions like heart disease. Studies show that the practice of Yoga lowers the cortisol levels, bringing a greater sense of calm and well-being.

5.5. Improving Coping Mechanisms and Healing Trauma

Restorative Yoga helps to improve the body's coping mechanisms and heals trauma. The practice involves focusing on the breath and the sensations arising in the body, helping increase body awareness and connectivity between the mind and body. This can be particularly beneficial in healing trauma and managing emotional responses to stressful situations.

Through Restorative Yoga, individuals learn to cultivate a non-reactive mind-set, managing their emotional responses rather than being overwhelmed by them. This practice brings greater mental clarity and peace, enabling the individual to respond to stressful situations more effectively.

To sum it up, the science behind Restorative Yoga underpins its efficacy in managing chronic illnesses and promoting holistic healing. Its therapeutic effects on the neurological, immune, and hormonal systems, coupled with its enhancement of coping mechanisms and trauma healing, provide strong evidence of its power as a tool for chronic illness management and overall wellness.

Through understanding the scientific mechanisms, we can approach Restorative Yoga with informed dedication, allowing us to unlock its full potential for healing and restoration.

Next, we delve into the anecdotal evidence, stories of triumph from those who regained health and vitality, further supporting the scientific foundations of Restorative Yoga. Indeed, Restorative Yoga might not just offer relief, but total wellness transformation.

Chapter 6. On Chronic Illness: A Broad Overview

In the contemporary health landscape, chronic illness is not an uncommon term. It punctuates nearly all forms of discourse - from health discussions at the family dinner table to global health conferences addressing pressing matters of public health. A chronic illness is typically characterized by its persistent and long-lasting effects, usually longer than three months. Chronic illnesses encompass a spectrum of conditions such as heart disease, diabetes, arthritis, mental illnesses, and multiple sclerosis, among others. These diseases impact millions globally and continue to form an increasing health burden, accompanied by serious psycho-social implications.

6.1. Understanding Chronic Illness

Profoundly, our understanding of chronic illness is often drawn from biomedical perspectives, primarily focusing on biological changes in bodily functions. In contrast, this biomedical model often shadows the intricacies of the experience of chronic illness, which extends well beyond medical descriptions or diagnostics. It includes a medley of physical discomfort, emotional distress, limitations on daily activities, and complexities of managing treatments. In essence, the ramifications of chronic illness are chaotic, disturbing the ebb and flow of life, dancing vigorously on the delicate cords of mental, physical, and social health.

Chronic illness tends to appear unexpectedly and might escalate gradually, silently, over extended periods before the first symptoms appear. The periodicity and intensity of the disease may vary. Some illnesses have periods of remission where there are no symptoms, while others persist consistently. The trajectory is unpredictable, disruptive, and often marked by a struggle to get a clear diagnosis and effective treatment.

6.2. Biopsychosocial Model of Chronic Illness

The biopsychosocial model offers a comprehensive approach to understand the causes and effects of chronic illness. This model underscores three major aspects inextricably linked: biological, psychological, and social factors.

The biological component refers to how the disease affects bodily functions and structures. Meanwhile, the psychological component enhances our understanding of emotional responses, mental health issues, cognitive changes, and coping mechanisms tied to illness experiences. Lastly, the social component examines how sociocultural factors like socio-economic status, culture, and social support contribute to the onset and progression of diseases, and how the disease impacts societal roles and relationships.

6.3. The Rising Prevalence of Chronic Illness

Chronic diseases have seen a dramatic rise in recent years, evident from worldwide statistics. The increasingly aging global population, urbanization, sedentary lifestyles, inadequate nutrition, and rising pollution are among the key factors contributing to this alarming escalation.

According to the World Health Organization, chronic diseases are projected to account for 73% of all deaths globally by 2020. In fact, chronic conditions such as heart disease, stroke, and diabetes are now leading causes of death and disability, signifying a paradigm shift from acute to chronic diseases in global health.

6.4. The Impact on Quality of Life

The profound impacts of chronic illnesses on quality of life should not be underestimated. Physical symptoms such as pain or fatigue can be debilitating, dramatically reducing functionality and independence. The financial strain of treatments, coupled with reduced earning capacity, can lead to significant stress. Furthermore, the emotional impacts - anxiety, depression, or feelings of hopelessness - add a hidden, yet profound dimension to the burdens of chronic disease. Equally crucial is the strain these conditions can place on relationships, disrupting personal and professional life to a remarkable extent.

Yet, there is a silver lining!

6.5. Hope Amid Desolation: The Transformative Power of Restorative Yoga

Restorative Yoga, as we shall explore in subsequent chapters, stands as a beacon of hope to those grappling with the implications of chronic illness. Mixing ancient yogic wisdom with modern science, this unique practice provides an oasis of calm in the tempestuous seas of chronic disease narratives.

By offering a sanctuary to reconnect with oneself, to breathe, and to find serenity amid chaos, Restorative Yoga enables healing on multiple levels - physical, mental, and spiritual. In the unfolding sections, we will embark on an expedition through the heart of this transformative practice, which has helped scores of chronic disease patients reclaim their lives, one mindful breath and pose at a time.

To conclude, chronic illnesses are more than just long-term medical conditions. They intertwine with numerous aspects of our lives, altering our perspectives on health and living. This chapter aimed to establish an understanding of these intertwined threads. Bearing in mind the complexities of chronic illness, we thus set the stage for the forthcoming exploration. Await the unveiling of the profound ways in which Restorative Yoga responds to these complexities, bringing rejuvenation, balance, and resilience even amid adversity and affliction.

Chapter 7. Impact of Restorative Yoga on Chronic Illness

In the vast expanse of therapeutic strategies for managing chronic illness, restorative yoga shines as an effective non-pharmacological intervention. Its subtle potency lies in its ability to address the diverse aspects of chronic diseases. By grounding and calming the practitioner, restorative yoga brings a symbiosis of bodily relaxation and mental serenity, which facilitates healing at multiple levels.

7.1. The Interplay of Stress and Chronic Illness

In understanding the power of restorative yoga, it is crucial to first consider the insidious role of stress in chronic conditions. Whether it be chronic pain syndromes, cardiovascular diseases, or autoimmune disorders, research consistently shows a link between stress and these ailments. Extended periods of stress skew the balance of the body's hormonal and nervous systems, fostering a dysfunctional immune system that creates an ideal environment for chronic diseases to thrive.

An alchemical formula of props, poses, and deep breathing, restorative yoga serves as an antidote to this problem. With its emphasis on parasympathetic nervous system activation, restorative yoga pulls back the throttle on the body's stress response, providing a route to wellness that conventional medicine often overlooks.

7.2. Parasympathetic Activation and Yoga

The parasympathetic nervous system is the part of the autonomic nervous system that helps the body 'rest and digest.' It slows the heart rate, lowers blood pressure, and redirects blood flow towards the internal organs, promoting their optimal functioning.

Restorative yoga encourages us to slow down and enter a relaxed state, activating the parasympathetic nervous system. As we sink into our props and surrender the weight of our bodies, the slow, rhythmic pattern of our breath signals safety to our nervous systems. This initiates the cascade of parasympathetic responses that counteract the harmful effects of chronic stress and illness.

7.3. Attend to the Breath

Breathing practices, or pranayama, are a cornerstone of restorative yoga. Pranayama is known to directly influence the autonomic nervous system, balancing the dyad of 'fight or flight' and 'rest and digest.' Several research studies demonstrate that regular practice of specific pranayama techniques reduces stress hormones, promotes heart rate variability (a marker of resilience), and improves lung function; all of which confer benefits for chronic illness patients.

7.4. From Asana to Relaxation

Restorative yoga poses, called asanas, are crafted to provide maximum comfort and minimum strain, allowing the practitioner to develop a deep awareness of the body. This awareness acts as a bridge to relaxation and healing by discouraging the harmful cycle of tension, discomfort and stress that underlies many chronic conditions. Each asana invokes a sense of grounding, reassurance and support, muscling a space for restoration and healing.

7.5. The Significant Role of Props

Props such as bolsters, blankets, and blocks are staples of restorative yoga. They provide a support system that allows one to stay in poses for extended periods, without the tension that often accompanies traditional yoga poses. The use of props produces a profound sense of security and stability, preventing harmful stress responses and promoting deep relaxation and healing.

7.6. Stories of Transformation

Numerous testimonials from individuals suffering from a variety of chronic illnesses demonstrate the far-reaching impact of restorative yoga. Ranging from stories of pain relief and enhanced mobility, to accounts of improved mood, better sleep, and increased energy, these narratives embody a practical and emotional testament to the therapeutic potency of restorative yoga.

To embody and encapsulate the wisdom within the world of restorative yoga necessitates total immersion. Give it a chance, and it could become an indispensable ally in your quest for well-being and resilience. This gentle practice, with its unique blend of bodily postures, breath control, and meditative awareness, stands as a beacon lighting the path to your body's natural potential for healing and harmony against the challenge of chronic disease.

Chapter 8. Testimonials: Stories of Triumph and Healing

When embarking on a journey towards healing, nothing speaks volumes like the testimonials of individuals who have walked this path before. In this chapter, we will traverse the landscapes of transformation, regaining health, and renewed vitality as we take you through real-life stories of triumph over chronic illnesses through Restorative Yoga.

8.1. A Beacon of Hope: Melissa's Story

Melissa's skirmish with chronic back pain started a decade ago. A slip-and-fall accident gave birth to an unwelcome guest that reigned over her life, triggering bouts of excruciating pain. Tired of living under a cloud of constant unease and discomfort, Melissa decided to explore alternative therapies and discovered Restorative Yoga. This was her turning point. Gentle poses guided her body to regain flexibility while the calm restored her sleep pattern. She soon realized that Restorative Yoga was far more than just a physical practice; it was her sanctuary, her defining journey back to health. Today, Melissa credits Restorative Yoga as her savior – for not just restoring her body's strength and flexibility but also reinstating her freedom from pain.

8.2. The Warrior Survivor: James' Journey

James' battle with chronic fatigue had been with him ever since his cancer diagnosis years ago. He recalls the aftermath of his treatments, how he felt drained, almost lifeless, in a void of endless fatigue. A fellow survivor introduced him to Restorative Yoga. Initially skeptical, he decided to give it a try. The first few sessions were physically challenging, but with every stretch and every breath, he felt a sense of release. Progress was slow and incremental, until one day, he awoke feeling rested and energized. This newfound vitality was not intoxicating; rather, it was soft, calm, and restorative. James found vitality in stillness, strength in surrender, and healing in tranquility.

8.3. Finding Peace in Pain: Sophia's Experience

Sophia was a chronic migraine sufferer. The pain persisted, unabated, ricocheting through her life like a wrecking ball. Frustrated and anxious, she sought out Restorative Yoga hoping to alleviate her discomfort. The practice opened pathways of calm, helping her manage anxiety and stress – known triggers for her migraines. Over time, the frequency and intensity of her headaches began to diminish. Routine practices led to a major shift — the pain no longer controlled her; she found acceptance and peace within her condition. Restorative Yoga taught her to sail smoothly over life's tumultuous waves. Today, Sophia's journey is an inspiration for others living with migraine, proving that, sometimes, dealing with pain may require repose and not war.

8.4. The Unseen Healer: Max's Progress

Depression had taken Max into its unfathomable depths. What was initially a low mood spiralled into a chronic condition. Seering loneliness and feelings of blunted self-worth clouded his perception. When medication and therapy were insufficient, he turned towards Restorative Yoga. Quiet, contemplative poses started to cultivate a compassionate dialogue with his body and mind. The practice served as a mirror, reflecting his own worth. Restorative Yoga became not only his physical practice but his mental release too. It provided him internal scaffolds to temper the turmoil inside. His loneliness took on a new form - solitude, a state where aloneness did not equate to emptiness. Max's story stands strong, demonstrating that healing is often an inside-out process; that in our quest for health, we often overlook the power within.

In these narratives, we journey through a terrain of healing piloted by courage, resilience, and acceptance. Each story stands as a testament to the transformative power of Restorative Yoga. Our protagonists, Melissa, James, Sophia, and Max, transmogrified their struggles with chronic conditions into stories of triumph, affirming the potential of this humble practice. Their experiences echo the beauty of Restorative Yoga, where each breath has the magic to heal, and every pose carries the weight of wellness. Healing belongs to those who believe in its power and seek solace within themselves by courageous exploration of their own capacities to recover and restore.

Chapter 9. Safety and Best Practices in Restorative Yoga

The recognition of safety protocols and the execution of best practices stand central to any physical activity or fitness regime, and Restorative Yoga is no exception. It demands focus, patience, and respect for one's own physical boundaries, making the domain of safety and best practice a crucial component. This chapter aims to dissect the nuances of ensuring a safe and fulfilling restorative yoga practice.

9.1. Identifying Personal Limitations

Everyone's body is unique, and it's essential to understand one's own personal limitations before diving into a restorative yoga practice. Consider any pre-existing conditions or injuries and how they may affect your yoga sessions. Remember, yoga, especially restorative yoga, is not about pushing your body to the limit; it's about healing, restoring, and rejuvenating in a calm and gentle manner.

9.2. The Role of a Qualified Instructor

In learning and practicing Restorative Yoga safely, a qualified instructor plays a guiding role. A knowledgeable teacher can help you achieve proper alignment, modify poses according to your needs, and prevent injury. They can also ensure that you are using yoga props correctly, a key element in Restorative Yoga. Signing up for classes with an experienced and certified teacher is highly advised.

9.3. Correct Use of Yoga Props

Restorative Yoga often utilizes props like bolsters, blankets, yoga blocks, and straps to help the body achieve and maintain different poses without strain. It's vital to understand how to use these props correctly to maximize their benefits and make your yoga practice safe and effective.

- **Bolsters**: These are typically used to provide support in poses enabling deep relaxation. Care should be taken to place them in a way that aligns the body properly, preventing overstretching or straining.

- **Blankets**: These can be used for comfort, warmth, and support in various poses. Always ensure the blanket is folded neatly to provide even support.

- **Yoga Blocks**: Blocks are used to bring the ground closer in poses where the hands aren't able to reach the floor easily. They can also provide support in seated and supine poses.

- **Yoga Straps**: Straps can be used to increase reach in poses where the hands cannot meet. They help maintain alignment and promote safe stretching.

9.4. Listening to Your Body: An Essential Practice

It's important to tune in and listen to the signals your body sends. If you feel pain or discomfort in a pose, it could be an indication that your body is being pushed too hard or a pose is not correct for you at that moment. Rather than pushing through the pain, try modifying the pose or using props for support.

9.5. Breathing: Pranayama Techniques

In the realm of yoga, breath control, known as Pranayama, is essential. It is instrumental in soothing the nervous system and ensuring internal steadiness. Particularly in restorative yoga, practitioners are urged to practice deep diaphragmatic breathing, promoting calmness and serving as an organic tool for resilience against stress. Adapting correct breathing techniques within and outside of the practice can significantly enhance the overall restorative yoga experience.

9.6. Importance of Warm-Up and Cool-Down

The act of warming up the body before starting restorative yoga is necessary, especially in colder weather. Simple warm-up exercises prepare your muscles and joints for the yoga session and reduce the risk of injuries. Similarly, cooling down after practice helps your body to gradually transition from the active yoga practice to your normal state.

9.7. Regular Practice: Consistency is Key

Regular practice is integral to safely improving your restorative yoga journey. Developing a consistent routine will gradually enhance your flexibility, strength, and understanding of the practice, reducing the risk of injury. However, remember that it's not about how often you practice, but rather the quality and attentiveness you bring into each session.

Restorative Yoga, while gentle, requires that attention be paid to the essentials of safety and best practices. This is particularly crucial for those managing chronic illnesses, but is equally important for those looking for a deeper, more mindful connection with their bodies.

Chapter 10. Getting Started with Restorative Yoga: A How-to Guide

Welcome to the entrancing world of Restorative Yoga. Before you begin your journey, let's understand what Restorative Yoga is and why it's a beneficial practice.

Restorative Yoga is a therapeutic style of Yoga that uses props to support the body, allowing it to fully relax while holding poses. It is characterized by long-held, passive postures intended to restore the body to its optimal health, balance, and vitality.

Restorative Yoga stands apart from the more vigorous styles of Yoga. It's about slowing down, settling into stillness, and letting the body naturally rejuvenate and heal. Each pose is designed not just to stretch your muscles but to harmonize the body, calm the mind, and heal the spirit.

10.1. Let's Get Started: Understanding The Basics

To get started, you will need comfortable clothing that allows your body to move freely. Yoga mats, blocks, bolsters, blankets, and straps are commonly used to support the body in various poses. Don't fret if you don't have these props - a firm pillow, a towel, and a scarf can be easily substituted.

The environment you choose is equally important. Choose a quiet place where you won't be disturbed. You may consider dimming the lights, playing soft music, and lighting a candle for a more calming atmosphere.

When practicing restorative yoga, it's crucial to listen to your body and its limits. If a pose doesn't feel right or causes pain, ease out of it gently. Remember, the goal is not to stretch as far as possible, but to find a place of comfort and stillness.

10.2. First Steps: Basic Restorative Yoga Poses

Restorative Yoga is designed to be accessible to everyone, regardless of age, ability, or flexibility. Here are a few fundamental restorative yoga poses to get you started.

1. **Child's Pose (Balasana):** This pose gently stretches the back, hips, thighs, and ankles while soothing the mind. Start on your hands and knees, with your big toes touching. Spread your knees apart and sit back on your heels. Extend your arms in front of you and place your forehead on your mat or a bolster.

2. **Supported Forward Bend (Paschimottanasana):** Seated on your mat, extend your legs in front of you. Place a bolster or pillow on your thighs. Gently bend forward from your hips, allowing your body to rest on the bolster. This pose stretches the spine and the back of your legs.

3. **Legs-Up-The-Wall Pose (Viparita Karani):** This pose releases tension in the legs and lower back. Place a bolster or blanket against a wall. Sit sideways on the bolster, then gently swing your legs up the wall as you lay down on your back. Let your arms rest by your sides.

10.3. Pacing Your Practice

When performing these poses, try to hold each pose for at least 5 minutes. Take deep, slow breaths, focusing on the rise and fall of your breath. As you exhale, allow tension to melt away from your body.

Adjust the props as needed to ensure you're comfortable in each pose. Comfort is key in Restorative Yoga - if you don't feel quite right, adjust the props, alter the pose or switch to a different pose altogether.

Remember that Restorative Yoga is meant to be a slow, calming practice. Don't rush through the poses; instead, enjoy each moment of stillness and relaxation.

10.4. Deepening Your Practice: Advanced Restorative Yoga Poses

Once you're comfortable with the basic poses, you may wish to explore more advanced restorative poses, such as Supported Bridge Pose (Setu Bandhasana), Reclining Hero Pose (Supta Virasana), and Supported Fish Pose (Matsyasana). These poses can help address specific areas of tension and imbalance in your body. However, always ensure your body is comfortable and supported.

At the heart of Restorative Yoga is the art of surrendering—a surrendering of our bodies to the pose, of our minds to the breath, and of our thoughts to stillness. Practicing Restorative Yoga is an open invitation to explore the limitless potential for healing, comfort, and balance that exists within each of us.

May your exploration of Restorative Yoga transform your life, just as it has transformed countless others. Let the journey begin.

Chapter 11. Restorative Yoga as a Lifestyle: Building Your Daily Practice

Adopting Restorative Yoga as a lifestyle implies transforming it from a mere physical exercise into an integral part of your daily activities. It means that this practice goes beyond your time on the mat, seeping into every facet of your life, reinforcing your overall wellbeing.

11.1. Embracing Yoga's Restorative Path

Yoga is an ancient practice with a rich heritage that has been passed down through generations. While various yoga styles focus on strength, flexibility, and balance, restorative yoga sets itself apart with its emphasis on relaxation and healing. It is a practice intentionally designed to invoke calm, reduce stress, and act as a counterpoint to our often overly-active lifestyles.

To truly adopt Restorative Yoga as a lifestyle, you need to understand its fundamental principles – relaxation, healing, and mindfulness. It requires an appreciation for slower flows, longer holds, and truly inhabiting each posture, somatically and mindfully connecting with your body in every pose. This gentle approach encourages a shift away from the hectic hustle of the everyday life, offering a reservoir of tranquility that you can tap into anytime and anywhere.

11.2. Starting Your Daily Routine

When starting a new habit, it's crucial to start modestly to avoid overwhelming yourself. Begin with a short, 15-minute session each morning. Try choosing one or two poses that you particularly enjoy and spend some time exploring them. As the routine becomes more ingrained and your comfort level increases, gradually extend your practice.

Here are some useful tips for creating a daily restorative yoga routine:

1. Choose a specific time and place: Routine is an ally for building a new habit. Consider what time of day works best for you (many people find morning or evening particularly effective).

2. Make it enjoyable: The practice should be something you look forward to, not a chore. Create a sense of ritual around your practice, maybe by making your practice space beautiful with plants, candles, or any other soothing aesthetics.

3. Keep it simple: Restorative yoga is about relaxing and healing, not challenging your flexibility or strength. Choose poses that you enjoy and feel comfortable in.

4. Consistency is key: Practicing regularly, even if for shorter periods, helps build the habit effectively.

11.3. Unfolding The Restorative Poses

Restorative yoga makes use of a variety of poses, with each having its unique benefits. Here, we touch upon some poses that progressively extend and deepen your practice.

1. Child's Pose (Balasana): This is a grounding pose that promotes calmness and reduces stress. It can help stretch your hips, thighs, and ankles while relaxing your spine.

2. Legs-Up-The-Wall Pose (Viparita Karani): This soothing, gentle inversion helps to alleviate headaches, boost energy, and relieve

lower back pain.

3. Reclining Bound Angle Pose (Supta Baddha Konasana): Opening the hips and the chest, this pose aids deeper breathing, promotes relaxation, and eases tension.

4. Corpse Pose (Savasana): Usually the final pose in a yoga session, this asana promotes relaxation and rejuvenation, calming the brain, relieving stress, and aiding in relieving mild depression.

Remember, the beauty of Restorative Yoga lies in exploring the interplay between ease and patience. It's not about striving or forcing, but about nurturing and accepting.

11.4. Incorporating Mindfulness and Breathing Techniques

Mindfulness is the heart and soul of Restorative Yoga, and it's a lifestyle of its own. It's about being present, attending to the here-and-now without judgment.

In addition, breathwork or Pranayama is a significant part of restorative yoga. Proper breathing can enhance the healing effects of each pose and assist in obtaining a more profound sense of relaxation.

A common technique is abdominal breathing or diaphragmatic breathing. It initiates inhalation from the diaphragm, filling the lower part of the lungs first, then the middle, and then the top. This practice slows the breath rate, maximizes oxygen uptake, and engenders a sense of rest and relaxation.

Combining mindfulness and pranayama with restorative poses enriches our journey towards a yoga-centric lifestyle. It adds dimension to the practice, empowering a broader perspective and ingraining an enriched sensibility that extends beyond the mat.

11.5. Overcoming Challenges and Sustaining the Practice

Switching to a yoga-centric lifestyle can come with its own set of challenges - inertia, time scarcity, or even physical difficulties. However, patience, persistence, and consistency can make these hurdles surmountable. Remember, the aim is not to perfect a pose but to imbibe the serenity and healing that each pose holds.

In time, your consistent endeavor will weave the restorative practice into the fabric of your life. It will become more than a routine - a sanctuary you return to, a healing oasis amidst the whirls of daily life. On this journey, you'll discover not just a practice but a lifestyle that nurtures, heals and revives - one breath, one pose at a time.

Restorative Yoga as a lifestyle integrates the practice into your daily experiences, fostering health, harmony, and resilience. Immersed in this journey, you'll find a vessel of tranquility, a resilient spirit, and a renewed vigor for life's every moment. This transformative journey towards a restorative lifestyle awaits – and it all starts with you. Remember, the journey is just as important – if not more so – than the destination. Every breath you take, every pose you make - is a step into the serene world of restorative yoga.